REHABILITATION MASTERY OF THE HAND AND UPPER EXTREMITY

A complete Guide to Optimal Healing, Function, and Independence

Ricardo L. Jason

Table of Contents

CHAPTER ONE 4
   The foundations 4
   An analysis of the upper limb . 9

CHAPTER TWO 15
   Conditions and Treatments .. 15

CHAPTER THREE 25
   Musculoskeletal Disorders ... 25

CHAPTER FOUR 38
   Neurological Disorders 38
   Neurogenic Pain in the Upper Extremities 45

CHAPTER FIVE 52
   Brachial Plexus injuries and spinal cord injuries 52
   Edema lymphatic 60

CHAPTER SIX 68

Techniques for Rehabilitation 68

CHAPTER SEVEN 76

Healing Wounds and Scar Management 76

Design and Development of the Program 83

CHAPTER EIGHT 92

Particular Aspects to Take Into Account in Rehabilitation 92

THE END 101

Please consider leaving us a review. Thank you

CHAPTER ONE
The foundations

Anatomy and Upper Extremity Kinesiology

Comprehending the anatomy and kinesiology of the upper extremities is essential for a number of professions, including sports science, physical therapy, medicine, and more. Now let's explore each section:

1.1 Anatomy of the Hand:

The hand is a complicated anatomical structure made up of blood arteries, tendons, ligaments, muscles, and nerves. It is made up of the phalanges (finger bones), metacarpals (palm bones), and carpals (wrist bones). Fine motor skills and complex movements like pinching and gripping are controlled by the hand muscles.

1.2 Anatomy of the Wrist:

The joint that joins the hand and forearm is called the wrist. It is made up of two rows of eight carpal bones. These bones are held together by ligaments, which permits flexibility and stability. Tendons that govern hand movements are also located in the wrist; they travel via a small tunnel known as the carpal tunnel.

1.3 Elbow Structure:

The arm may be bent and straightened thanks to the elbow joint. The humerus (upper arm bone), radius, and ulna (forearm bone) make up its three bones. The tendons and ligaments that surround the elbow allow for mobility and stability.

Shoulder Anatomy (1.4):

The humerus and scapula (shoulder blade) combine to produce the shoulder, which is a ball-and-socket joint. Although it has a large range of motion, it is essentially unstable. The shoulder joint's supporting muscles, tendons, and ligaments cooperate to provide stability and enable actions like lifting, rotating, and reaching.

1.5 Upper Extremity Kinesiology:

Human movement is the subject of kinesiology. Analyzing the interplay between bones, muscles, and joints during different activities is essential to understanding the kinesiology of the upper extremities. The way the upper extremity performs actions like reaching, gripping, throwing, and lifting is influenced by a number of factors, including muscle strength, flexibility, coordination, and biomechanics.

It is imperative to have a comprehensive grasp of the anatomy and kinesiology of the upper extremities in order to diagnose and treat injuries, create rehabilitation plans, maximize athletic performance, and support musculoskeletal health in general.

An analysis of the upper limb

A thorough approach that includes collecting a history, doing a physical examination, and ordering diagnostic testing is required when examining the upper extremities. Let's examine each part in turn:

2.1 Recording History:

Taking a patient's history entails learning about their symptoms, health history, and any pertinent events that might have influenced their condition. Specific inquiries concerning the upper extremities could be:

Beginning and length of the symptoms

Type of pain (such as throbbing, dull, or severe)

Where the discomfort or agony is

Any past history of upper limb injuries or damage

Previous upper extremity-related illnesses or procedures

Any motions or activities that make symptoms worse or better

Any upper limb weakness, tingling, or numbness

2.2 Physical Assessment:

Assessing the range of motion, strength, sensitivity, and stability of the shoulder, elbow, wrist, and hand is part of a physical examination of the upper extremities. Important elements of the physical assessment could consist of:

Examining the upper limb for abnormalities, bruises, edema, or imbalance

palpation of particular anatomical landmarks, muscles, tendons, and ligaments to feel for anomalies or soreness

Range of motion evaluation for the fingers, wrist, elbow, and shoulder

Using physical muscle testing and resisted motions, one can assess the strength and integrity of muscles.

Sensation assessment by measurements of proprioception, light touch, and pinprick reactions

Evaluation of joint stability using specialist tests, such as the Lachman test for elbow stability and the Apprehension test for shoulder instability

2.3 Exams for Diagnosis:

To further assess the upper extremities and confirm or rule out particular disorders, diagnostic tests may be used. Typical diagnostic examinations consist of:

X-rays: Helpful in identifying degenerative changes in the bones and joints as well as fractures and dislocations.

Magnetic Resonance Imaging (MRI): This diagnostic tool can be used to identify soft tissue problems such rotator cuff tears or carpal tunnel syndrome. It produces detailed images of soft tissues, including muscles, tendons, ligaments...

Nerve conduction studies (NCS) and electromyography (EMG) are used to evaluate nerve function and diagnose diseases such peripheral neuropathy and nerve compression syndromes.

Ultrasound: Can be used to guide injections or screen for tendon disease. It can also be utilized to view soft tissue structures like ligaments and tendons.

Healthcare professionals can accurately diagnose disorders affecting the upper extremities and create a treatment plan by combining history taking, physical examination, and diagnostic testing.

CHAPTER TWO
Conditions and Treatments
Fractures and Dislocations

Breaks and Displacements

3.1 Broken Hand Bones:

Any of the several hand bones, such as the phalanges and metacarpals, might be fractured.

Depending on the location and severity of the fracture, treatment options include surgical fixation with pins, plates, or screws, closed reduction (manipulation of the fracture without surgery), and immobilization with splints or casts.

3.2 Broken Wrist Bones:

The ulna, carpal bones, and distal radius are frequently fractured in wrist fractures.

For stable fractures, treatment options include splinting or casting; for unstable fractures, surgical intervention such as open reduction and internal fixation (ORIF) with plates and screws may be necessary.

3.3 Broken Elbow Bones:

The proximal radius, ulna, or distal humerus can all be affected by elbow fractures.

Treatment options include closed reduction, surgical fixation with plates and screws, or immobilization with a cast or splint, depending on the kind and severity of the fracture.

3.4.1 Shoulder Fractures:

Shoulder fractures can affect the scapula, proximal humerus, or clavicle (collarbone).

Depending on the fracture's location and severity, different treatment options may be used, such as immobilization, closed reduction, or surgery with fixation devices.

3.5 Traumatic Upper Extremity Dislocations:

When a joint's bones are pushed out of their natural places, dislocations happen.

The most frequent dislocations of the upper extremities are those of the shoulder, elbow, and fingers.

Reducing the dislocated joint to its original position is the first step in treatment. After that, the joint is immobilized and therapy is performed to restore strength and range of motion. Surgical intervention might be required in certain instances to heal soft tissue or ligament damage.

It is crucial to treat upper extremity fractures and dislocations promptly and appropriately to avoid consequences such joint stiffness, nerve damage, and long-term functional impairment. To achieve the best possible results and speed up recovery, treatment plans should be customized for each patient's unique circumstances and the particular injury.

Soft Tissue Damage

Soft Tissue Damage

4.1 Bends and Twists:

The fibrous structures called ligaments, which attach bones to one another, can rip or stretch when a sprain occurs.

The elbow, wrist, fingers, and shoulder are among the upper extremity joints that are frequently impacted.

RICE (rest, ice, compression, and elevation) is the standard treatment plan, which also includes braces or splints to immobilize the patient. In order to regain range of motion and strength, physical therapy may be recommended.

Strains occur when tendons or muscles that attach muscles to bones are torn or stretched.

Similar to sprains, treatment entails rest, ice, compression, and elevation. Gradually increasing exercise and stretching are then used to help the injured muscle or tendon heal.

4.2 Tendon injuries and lacerations: Cuts or rips in the skin, commonly brought on by trauma or sharp instruments, are called lacerations.

In order to promote healing and prevent infection, treatment include thoroughly cleansing the wound, closing it with sutures or staples if needed, and applying dressings.

Mild tendonitis, or inflammation of the tendon, can be as severe as whole tendon rips.

Depending on how severe the injury is, the course of treatment may involve physical therapy, immobilization, rest, and in certain situations, surgery to heal the damage.

4.3 Burns:

Exposure to radiation, heat, chemicals, or electricity can all cause burns on the upper extremities.

Initially, the burn must be cooled with water. Then, the wound must be cleaned and dressed to stop infection. A burn center may be necessary for the treatment of severe burns.

Using physical therapy and occupational therapy, rehabilitation aims to preserve range of motion, avoid contractures (abnormal shortening of muscles and tendons), and maximize functional results.

The intricacy and severity of soft tissue injuries in the upper extremities can differ greatly. In order to reduce problems and promote the best possible recovery, prompt evaluation and appropriate management are crucial. Individualized treatment plans should take into account the patient's overall health, functional goals, and the kind and extent of the injury.

CHAPTER THREE
Musculoskeletal Disorders

Conditions Associated with Arthritis

Diabetic arthritis:

An inflammatory disease called rheumatoid arthritis (RA) is characterized by persistent joint inflammation, which can cause pain, swelling, stiffness, and eventually joint destruction.

Larger joints like the shoulders, elbows, and knees may also be affected, however it usually affects the little joints in the hands and feet.

Physical therapy, lifestyle changes, and pharmaceuticals (such as biologic agents and disease-modifying antirheumatic drugs) are used in combination to treat the condition with the goals of reducing inflammation, relieving pain, and maintaining joint function.

In extreme situations, pain relief and improved mobility may require surgical procedures such joint replacement surgery.

Osteoarthritis:

Osteoarthritis (OA) is a degenerative joint disease that causes pain, stiffness, and loss of motion due to the breakdown of cartilage in the joints.

It can also occur in the hands, wrists, and other joints of the upper extremities, but it usually affects weight-bearing joints like the knees, hips, and spine.

The goal of treatment is to improve joint function and manage symptoms by combining pharmaceuticals (like analgesics and nonsteroidal anti-inflammatory medicines) with non-pharmacological therapies (like physical therapy, exercise, and weight management).

In more severe situations, arthroscopic treatments or joint replacement surgery may be taken into consideration as surgical options to reduce discomfort and enhance function.

Additional Arthritic Disorders:

Additional arthritic conditions could be:

Those who have psoriasis may develop psoriatic arthritis, which can affect the joints, skin, and nails.

Ankylosing spondylitis is an inflammatory arthritis that mainly affects the sacroiliac and vertebral bodies, although it can also affect the hips, shoulders, and palms of the hands.

Gout is a type of arthritis that primarily affects the big toe but can also strike the hands and wrists. It is brought on by an accumulation of uric acid crystals in the joints.

Depending on the particular kind of arthritis, treatment for these disorders can involve a mix of drugs, physical therapy, lifestyle changes, and in certain situations, surgery.

Physical therapists, orthopedic surgeons, rheumatologists, and other medical specialists must collaborate to manage arthritis and associated disorders in the upper extremities. Reducing pain, enhancing joint function, and improving the quality of life for those with these persistent musculoskeletal conditions are the main objectives.

Combined Trauma Conditions

Cumulative trauma disorders (CTDs), sometimes referred to as overuse injuries or repetitive strain injuries (RSIs), are a collection of ailments brought on over time by severe exertions, uncomfortable postures, or repeated or prolonged motions. The muscles, tendons, ligaments, nerves, and other soft tissues in the body are the main targets of these illnesses. When it comes to the upper limb, CTDs typically affect the elbows, shoulders, hands, and wrists. CTDs affecting the upper extremities include, for instance:

Carpal Tunnel Syndrome:
Compression of the median nerve as it travels through the carpal tunnel in the wrist is the hallmark

of carpal tunnel syndrome, a frequent CTD.

Pain, tingling, numbness, and weakness in the hand are possible symptoms, especially in the thumb, index finger, middle finger, and half of the ring finger.

Uncomfortable hand positions, repetitive hand and wrist motions, and underlying medical disorders including diabetes or arthritis are risk factors.

(Lateral Epicondylitis): Tennis elbow

A CTD known as tennis elbow is typified by inflammation or

deterioration of the tendons that join the elbow's lateral epicondyle.

The condition usually manifests as discomfort and pain on the outside of the elbow, which might extend down the forearm.

Tennis, painting, and typing are a few examples of repetitive wrist extension or grasping activities that might exacerbate this disease.

Golfer's elbow, also known as medial epicondylitis:

Tennis elbow and golfer's elbow are similar in that they both affect the tendons that join to the medial epicondyle on the inside of the elbow.

Activities like lifting, golfing, or using hand tools that require gripping or repetitive wrist flexion can exacerbate it and produce pain and tenderness on the inside of the elbow.

Tennis elbow tendinitis:

A CTD that affects the muscles and tendons surrounding the shoulder joint is rotator cuff tendinitis.

It manifests as shoulder soreness and weakness, especially when reaching behind the back or overhead.

Muscle imbalances, bad posture, and repetitive shoulder motions are risk factors.

Tenosynovitis de Quervain:

An inflammatory condition affecting the tendons and their sheaths near the base of the thumb is known as De Quervain's tenosynovitis (CTD).

It results in pain, edema, and trouble moving the thumb and wrist, especially while doing tasks that need gripping or pinching actions.

Intervention and Prophylaxis:

Rest, activity modification, physical therapy, ergonomic measures, and occasionally bracing or splinting are the usual methods used in the management of CTDs.

Preventive measures include adopting ergonomic tools and equipment, taking regular breaks, stretching and strengthening exercises, and maintaining good posture.

For CTDs to not worsen and result in persistent pain or impairment, early detection and treatment are crucial.

People can prevent cumulative trauma disorders in the upper extremities and preserve musculoskeletal health by being aware of the risk factors, symptoms, and management of these conditions, particularly in occupations or activities that require repetitive or strenuous movements.

CHAPTER FOUR
Neurological Disorders
Damage to Peripheral Nerves

Disorders of the nervous system

Damage to Peripheral Nerves

Carpal Tunnel Syndrome:

A frequent peripheral nerve compression condition called carpal tunnel syndrome (CTS) is characterized by compression of the median nerve as it travels through the wrist's carpal tunnel.

Specifically in the thumb, index finger, middle finger, and half of the ring finger, the symptoms include discomfort, numbness, tingling, and weakness in the hand.

In cases with severe or resistant symptoms, treatment options range from conservative methods such as wrist splinting, corticosteroid injections, and ergonomic adjustments to surgical intervention.

Additional Syndromes of Nerve Compression:

The following are possible additional upper extremity nerve compression syndromes:

Cubital tunnel syndrome is characterized by ulnar nerve compression in the elbow, resulting in ring and little finger numbness, tingling, and weakness.

Compression of the radial nerve as it travels through the forearm causes radial tunnel syndrome, which is characterized by pain and weakness in the hand and forearm.

Compression of the nerves and blood vessels as they pass through the thoracic outlet causes thoracic outlet syndrome, which manifests as discomfort, numbness, and weakness in the hand, arm, and shoulder.

Damage to the Nerves:

Numerous injuries, such as cuts, fractures, dislocations, and crush injuries, can induce traumatic nerve damage in the upper extremities.

Pain, numbness, weakness, and loss of sensation or motor function are examples of symptoms that can result from partial or total disruption of nerve function, depending on the extent and location of the damage.

To restore nerve continuity and function, treatment options include nerve transfer, nerve grafting, and surgical repair. To maximize recovery and restore function, rehabilitation, which includes physical therapy and occupational therapy, is frequently required.

Identification and Handling:

Peripheral nerve injuries are diagnosed with a comprehensive history, physical examination, and frequently electrodiagnostic tests including electromyography and nerve conduction investigations.

The precise nerve implicated, the extent of the damage, and the objectives and preferences of each patient all influence the management techniques.

In order to minimize consequences and avoid irreversible nerve injury, early detection and treatment are essential. For a thorough assessment and treatment of peripheral nerve problems in the upper extremities, multidisciplinary care involving neurologists, orthopedic surgeons, hand surgeons, and rehabilitation specialists is sometimes required. Healthcare professionals who treat patients with neurological illnesses affecting the hand, wrist, elbow, and shoulder must be knowledgeable with the presentation, diagnosis, and treatment of compression syndromes and peripheral nerve injuries in the upper extremities.

Neurogenic Pain in the Upper Extremities

9.1 CRPS, or complex regional pain syndrome:

Previously known as causalgia or reflex sympathetic dystrophy (RSD), complex regional pain syndrome (CRPS) is a persistent pain condition that usually affects one limb, frequently following surgery or trauma.

Severe burning pain, edema, temperature and color changes in the skin, and extreme sensitivity to cold or touch are its characteristic symptoms.

It is thought that CRPS is caused by malfunctions in the peripheral and central neurological systems, which result in aberrant inflammation and pain signals.

A multidisciplinary approach to treatment may involve drugs (such as antidepressants, bisphosphonates, analgesics, or anticonvulsants), occupational therapy, physical therapy, spinal cord stimulation, nerve blocks, or other interventional treatments in addition to physical therapy and occupational therapy. Counseling and psychosocial support could be helpful as well.

9.2 Additional Painful Illnesses:

Other excruciating ailments that could impact the upper limbs include:

Trauma, tumors, or compression can cause damage to the brachial plexus, which can cause excruciating pain, weakness, and abnormal sensation in the hand, arm, and shoulder.

Peripheral neuropathy, radiculopathy, and nerve entrapment syndromes are examples of neuropathic pain syndromes that can produce burning or shooting pain, tingling, numbness, or weakness in the upper extremities.

Myofascial pain syndrome is a condition marked by trigger points or overuse-related localized muscle soreness and pain.

Compression of the nerves and blood vessels as they pass through the thoracic outlet causes thoracic outlet syndrome, which causes discomfort, numbness, and weakness in the hand, arm, and shoulder.

In order to address the underlying cause or relieve symptoms, treatment for these diseases may involve a mix of drugs, physical therapy, nerve blocks, injections, and, in certain situations, surgical intervention.

Identification and Handling:

When diagnosing neurogenic pain disorders in the upper extremities, a thorough evaluation is conducted. This includes a thorough history, a physical examination, and occasionally diagnostic testing such nerve conduction studies, electromyography, imaging investigations, or diagnostic nerve blocks.

Management options use a multimodal approach customized to each patient's needs and goals in an effort to reduce pain, increase function, and improve quality of life.

In order to effectively address the complicated nature of these disorders, teamwork among healthcare specialists from multiple specialties, such as pain medicine, neurology, orthopedic surgery, physical therapy, and psychiatry, may be necessary.

Healthcare professionals who are involved in the care of patients with chronic pain affecting the hand, wrist, elbow, and shoulder must have a thorough understanding of the presentation, diagnosis, and therapy of upper extremity neurogenic pain syndromes. People who live with these difficult disorders can experience better outcomes and less suffering if they receive early detection and assistance.

CHAPTER FIVE
Brachial Plexus injuries and spinal cord injuries

SCI, or spinal cord injury:

Synopsis:

Damage to the spinal cord that results in loss of motor, sensory, and autonomic function below the level of injury is referred to as spinal cord injury (SCI).

Traumatic injuries (from car crashes, falls, or sports injuries) and non-traumatic illnesses (from tumors, infections, or degenerative diseases) are among the causes of spinal cord injury (SCI).

The degree and completeness of the injury determine the severity and breadth of disability; more severe injuries lead to more widespread deficiencies.

Signs and Consequences:

SCI symptoms might include weakness or paralysis, loss of feeling, changes in bowel and bladder function, difficulties breathing, and even autonomic dysfunction.

Pressure ulcers, UTIs, respiratory issues, stiffness, neuropathic pain, and psychosocial difficulties are among the problems linked to SCI.

Identification and Handling:

A comprehensive neurological examination, imaging tests (such as MRIs, CT scans, or X-rays), and evaluation of sensory and motor function are all necessary for the diagnosis of SCI.

Preventing more damage, maintaining spinal stability, controlling complications, and encouraging functional recovery and rehabilitation are the main goals of managing scoli.

Spinal stabilization surgery, pain, spasticity, and neuropathic pain management drugs, assistive technology, psychological support, and rehabilitation therapy (physical, occupational, and speech therapy) are some of the possible course of treatment.

Trauma to the Brachial Plexus:

Synopsis:

The nerve network that regulates sensation and movement in the hand, arm, and shoulder is known as the brachial plexus.

Brachial plexus injuries are caused by trauma or stretching of the brachial plexus nerves, which results in loss of function, numbness, and weakness in the affected limb.

Automobile accidents, sports injuries, falls, and obstetric injuries sustained after childbirth are among the causes of brachial plexus injuries.

Brachial Plexus Injury Types:

Various types of brachial plexus injuries can be distinguished according to the extent and location of the injury, such as:

Neurapraxia: A brief loss of nerve function brought on by stretching or compression without causing structural nerve damage.

Axonotmesis: Damage to the nerve fibers that causes a loss of function, either permanent or temporary.

Complete nerve disruption, known as neurotmesis, necessitating grafting or surgical repair.

Identification and Handling:

A complete physical examination, evaluation of motor and sensory function, and diagnostic procedures including nerve conduction studies and electromyography (EMG) are all necessary for the diagnosis of brachial plexus injuries.

Treatment options for brachial plexus injuries range from

conservative methods (physical therapy, occupational therapy) to surgical intervention (nerve repair, nerve grafting, or nerve transfer procedures). The management of these injuries relies on the kind and degree of the damage.

The degree of nerve injury, the timing of intervention, and the success of rehabilitation efforts all influence the recovery prognosis.

Caretakers of patients with traumatic or non-traumatic injuries affecting the upper extremities and neurological function must have a thorough understanding of the traits, causes, diagnosis, and treatment of brachial plexus injuries and spinal cord injuries. For those with these difficult disorders, early identification, suitable intervention, and thorough rehabilitation are essential to maximizing results and raising quality of life.

Edema lymphatic
Additional Requirements

edema lymphatica:

Chronic lymphedema is characterized by swelling (edema) brought on by a build-up of lymphatic fluid in the tissues. It usually happens when lymphatic drainage is compromised due to damage, blockage, or removal of lymphatic vessels. Radiation therapy, infection, trauma, congenital abnormalities, and surgery (e.g., lymph node dissection for cancer treatment) can all cause lymphedema in the upper extremities.

Identification and Handling:

The clinical evaluation, which includes measurements of the limb circumference, tissue texture, and the existence of pitting edema, is the basis for the diagnosis. It is possible to evaluate lymphatic function with imaging tests like lymphoscintigraphy.

The objectives of lymphedema management are to lessen swelling, enhance lymphatic outflow, and avoid complications. Manual lymphatic drainage, compression therapy (bandaging or wearing compression garments), physical activity, skin care, and pneumatic compression devices are among possible treatment options. Surgical procedures like lymph node transfer or lymphaticovenous anastomosis may be explored in specific situations.

Birth Defects and Limb Losses:

Upper extremity congenital anomalies are defined as anatomical defects that exist from birth and can impact the blood vessels, muscles, tendons, bones, or nerves. Syndactyly (fused fingers), brachydactyly (short fingers), polydactyly (additional fingers), and radial club hand (malformation of the thumb and radius) are a few examples. Depending on the particular deformity, treatment options include prosthetic devices, surgical correction, or adaptive measures to enhance look and function.

Tumors, vascular disorders, congenital anomalies, and severe injuries can all lead to upper extremity amputations. Amputations of the upper limb can significantly affect a person's physical, functional, and mental health. Optimizing residual limb function, regaining mobility, and easing the use of prosthetic devices to improve independence and quality of life are the main goals of rehabilitation after amputation.

Skin and Nail Conditions:
The upper extremity can be impacted by a number of skin and nail diseases, including:
Psoriasis and dermatitis (eczema) can result in skin inflammation, scaling, redness, and itching.

Contact dermatitis, which causes blistering or a localized rash after being exposed to irritants or allergens.

Athlete's foot and ringworm are examples of fungal diseases that can affect the skin and nails, producing itching, redness, and nail thickening.

Changes in nail color, texture, or shape are indicative of nail disorders (onychomycosis), which are frequently brought on by fungus infections, injuries, or systemic illnesses.

Depending on the underlying reason, treatment for upper extremity skin and nail disorders can vary and may involve topical or oral drugs, antifungal therapies, moisturizers, corticosteroids, and lifestyle changes to lessen triggers or aggravating factors.

A multidisciplinary approach involving healthcare professionals from different specialties, such as rehabilitation medicine, orthopedics, plastic surgery, dermatology, and occupational therapy, is necessary to comprehend and manage lymphedema, congenital anomalies, amputations, and skin/nail conditions in the upper extremities. Personalized interventions and all-encompassing care plans are necessary to meet the special requirements and difficulties faced by people with these illnesses.

CHAPTER SIX
Techniques for Rehabilitation

Therapeutic Approaches:

Non-invasive treatments called "therapeutic modalities" are employed to lessen discomfort and inflammation while accelerating tissue repair. In upper extremity rehabilitation, common modalities include:

Heat therapy is the use of heat (such as hot packs or warm spa baths) to treat pain and stiffness, relax muscles, and improve blood flow.

Cold therapy is the application of cold (ice packs, cold compresses, etc.) to lessen pain, inflammation, and spasms in the muscles.

Electrical stimulation is the application of electrical currents to activate muscles and nerves, encourage contractions of the muscles, enhance blood flow, and control pain. Neuromuscular electrical stimulation (NMES) and transcutaneous electrical nerve stimulation (TENS) are two examples.

High-frequency sound waves are used in ultrasound therapy to warm deep tissue, improve blood flow, and encourage tissue repair.

Iontophoresis: The application of a low-level electrical current to the skin to deliver medication, such as anti-inflammatory medications.

Rehabilitative Exercise:

Enhancing upper extremity strength, flexibility, endurance, and functional ability is mostly dependent on therapeutic exercise. Activities could be:

Exercises for Range of Motion (ROM): Passive or active motions to increase joint flexibility and mobility.

Strengthening exercises involve resistance training to build muscle endurance and strength utilizing weights, resistance bands, or body weight.

Exercises that test proprioception, balance, and coordination in order to improve joint stability and control are known as proprioceptive exercises.

Functional training consists of exercises that mimic real-world tasks in order to enhance particular functional skills, like reaching, gripping, and object manipulation.

Manual Therapy Methods:

Manual therapy methods include manipulating soft tissues and joints with the hands in order to increase range of motion, lessen discomfort, and regain function. As examples, consider:

Soft Tissue Mobilization: Methods to relax stress, increase blood flow, and lessen muscle contraction, such as massage, myofascial release, and trigger point therapy.

Joint mobilization is the process of gently moving the joints in order to ease pain, lessen stiffness, and restore normal joint mechanics.

Manual stretching: Methods to increase flexibility, lengthen muscles and connective tissues, and lessen adhesions or contractures.

Orthotics and Assistive Technologies:

Orthotics and assistive technology are tools made to protect, support, or improve upper extremity function. As examples, consider:

Orthoses are braces, splints, or supports that are either custom-made or readily available and are used to stabilize joints, adjust alignment, or stop abnormalities.

Artificial limbs or portions intended to replace amputated or missing upper extremity parts, such as hands, fingers, or arms, are known as prosthetic devices.

Adaptive equipment refers to tools, utensils, or gadgets with altered designs or ergonomic elements that help with activities of daily living (ADLs) including getting dressed, taking care of oneself, cooking, or operating a vehicle.

Upper extremity rehabilitation procedures are designed to treat impairments, restore function, and enhance the quality of life for those who have functional, neurological, or musculoskeletal restrictions. Depending on the unique requirements and objectives of every patient, a complete rehabilitation program may combine manual treatment methods, therapeutic exercise, therapeutic modalities, and assistive technology. To get the best results and maximum recovery, healthcare professionals—physical therapists, occupational therapists, orthopedic surgeons, and rehabilitation specialists—must work together.

CHAPTER SEVEN
Healing Wounds and Scar Management

The Healing Process of Wounds:

The biological process of wound healing is intricate and involves multiple overlapping stages.

Hemostasis: Platelets clump together to halt the bleeding, and blood arteries narrow to lessen the bleeding.

Inflammatory Phase: To aid in healing, inflammatory cytokines trigger immune cell migration while white blood cells clear bacteria and debris from the wound site.

Proliferative Phase: Angiogenesis, the growth of blood vessels, supplies oxygen and nutrition as new tissue (granulation tissue) fills up the wound. Collagen is created by fibroblasts, fortifying the wound.

Phase of Remodeling: Scar development occurs as a result of collagen fibers maturing and rearranging within the wound. The scar could get flatter, softer, and less visible over time.

Scar Management:

The goals of effective scar treatment are to reduce scar development and maximize wound healing. Some possible strategies are as follows:

Wound Care: For the best chance of healing, the wound must be kept clean, moist, and free from infections. This could entail doing a light wash with warm water and soap, using bandages or antibiotic ointments, and avoiding activities that could agitate the wound.

Scar Massage: Using hydrating lotions or oils, massage the scar tissue to help soften the scar, increase blood flow, and lessen adhesions. To encourage flexibility and mobility, the scar should be massaged several times a day with light, circular motions.

Silicone Gel or Sheets: By moisturizing the skin, lowering inflammation, and enhancing the appearance of scars, silicone treatments are frequently used to manage scars. To smooth and flatten the scar, silicone gel or sheets are placed directly to the area and worn for a few hours each day.

Compression therapy: Applying pressure to the scar with bandages or compression garments can reduce swelling and encourage collagen alignment. This can lessen the likelihood of keloid or hypertrophic scarring, particularly in tension-prone areas.

Topical Treatments: To reduce scar inflammation and discolouration, a variety of topical treatments can be applied, including topical steroids, vitamin E, and onion extract (available in products like Mederma). However, each person will respond differently, and their effectiveness varies.

Scar Revision Surgery: Surgical intervention may be undertaken to improve the appearance or function of a scar that is conspicuous or functionally restrictive. Techniques include tissue reorganization, laser therapy, and scar excision.

Avoidance:

The first step in preventing severe scarring is to properly manage and care for wounds during the initial healing phase. Certain strategies can help promote favorable wound healing and lower the risk of aberrant scarring. These strategies include limiting tissue stress, avoiding strain on the wound margins, and optimizing nutrition and hydration.

Multidisciplinary Method:

A multidisciplinary strategy comprising medical specialists such wound care specialists, plastic surgeons, dermatologists, and physical therapists is frequently necessary for scar management. Customized treatment regimens should be created based on the unique features of the wound as well as the patient's preferences and objectives. Continuous monitoring and revisions should be made as necessary to maximize results.

Design and Development of the Program

Program Structure and Advancement for Rehabilitation of the Upper Extremities

Developing a structured strategy that is adapted to each patient's unique needs, objectives, and capabilities is a crucial step in designing an upper extremity rehabilitation program. Restoring function, lowering discomfort, increasing mobility, and improving quality of life should all be goals of the program. The following are essential elements to take into account when creating and **developing a rehabilitation program:**

1. First Evaluation:

Examine the patient's medical history, functional restrictions, impairments, and objectives in detail.

To create baseline data, assess range of motion, strength, feeling, and functional abilities objectively.

2. Establishing Objectives:

Work together with the patient to create both short- and long-term goals that are reasonable and doable.

Objectives ought to be SMART (specific, measurable, achievable, relevant, and time-bound), taking into account the patient's priorities and intended results.

3. Planning for Treatment:

Create a customized treatment plan based on the objectives and results of the assessment.

When applicable, take into account using manual therapy techniques, therapeutic exercises, therapeutic modalities, and assistive technology.

4. Exercise Guidelines:

To correct deficiencies in proprioception, strength, flexibility, and range of motion, prescribe therapeutic activities.

Exercises should be advanced progressively in terms of length, difficulty, and intensity to challenge the patient and reduce the chance of harm.

5. Hand Therapy:

To increase tissue flexibility, joint mobility, and pain alleviation, incorporate manual therapy techniques such soft tissue mobilization, joint mobilization, and manual stretching.

6. Therapeutic Approaches:

As an addition to physical therapy and exercise, employ therapeutic modalities like heat, cold, electrical stimulation, ultrasound, and iontophoresis to lessen pain, enhance tissue healing, and reduce inflammation.

7. Learning and Self-Control:

Instruct patients on appropriate body mechanics, ergonomic practices, and at-home workout regimens to enable them to actively participate in their recovery.

To encourage long-term self-management and independence,

teach pain management, activity moderation, and injury prevention techniques.

8. Advancement:

Regularly assess the patient's progress and modify the treatment plan in response to objective data and patient input.

As the patient gets better, progressively increase the level of difficulty, frequency, and complexity of the exercises and activities to make sure the program is both demanding and doable.

9. Practical Instruction:

Include tasks and functional activities that are pertinent to the patient's everyday activities and goals.

To make sure the patient can apply their skills and talents in real-world contexts, use realistic scenarios to imitate occupational tasks and activities of daily living (ADLs).

10. Review of goals and reevaluation:

Reevaluate the patient's functional results and progress on a regular basis to determine how well the rehabilitation program worked.

As the patient's condition changes or new priorities arise, modify your treatment plan and goals accordingly.

Healthcare practitioners can improve outcomes and speed up the rehabilitation process for patients with upper extremity injuries or diseases by designing and implementing programs with a thorough and methodical approach. Successful rehabilitation programs emphasize effective communication, teamwork, and patient engagement as essential elements that encourage empowerment and active participation throughout the healing process.

CHAPTER EIGHT
Particular Aspects to Take Into Account in Rehabilitation

Rehabilitation for Children:

The goals of pediatric rehabilitation are to maximize function and foster independence in kids who have injuries, developmental delays, or congenital or acquired disabilities. In pediatric rehabilitation, some things to keep in mind are:

Developmental Stage: Adapt interventions to the skills, interests, and developmental stage of the kid. Engage children in treatment through age-appropriate exercises and play-based activities.

Family-Centered Care: Include family members, parents, and caregivers in the healing process. To enable families to take an active role in their child's care and to speak out for their needs, provide them with information, resources, and support.

Interdisciplinary Approach: To fully address the complex needs of pediatric patients, work in conjunction with a multidisciplinary team that includes educators, psychologists, occupational therapists, physical therapists, and speech therapists.

Early Intervention: In order to maximize results in pediatric rehabilitation, early detection and intervention are essential. Provide early intervention treatments to improve motor skills, address developmental delays, and improve functional abilities from birth.

Senior Rehabilitation:

The goal of geriatric rehabilitation is to help older persons with age-related impairments, chronic conditions, or disabilities maintain or improve their function, mobility, and quality of life. **A few things to think about in geriatric rehabilitation are:**

Multimorbidity: Complex medical issues and numerous comorbidities are common in older persons. In order to fully attend to the patient's medical needs, coordinate care with specialists, general practitioners, and other healthcare professionals.

Fall Prevention: Serious injuries and a decline in functional abilities can result from falls, which is a major worry for older persons. Put into practice fall prevention techniques, such as strength training, house modifications, balance training, and fall risk education.

Cognitive Impairment: During rehabilitation, take care of issues relating to dementia and cognitive impairment. Modify treatment strategies, offer memory aids, and include caregivers in helping the patient maintain their functional and cognitive capacities.

Polypharmacy: The risk of negative drug responses and interactions is increased in older persons who may be taking many drugs. Work together to review prescriptions, reduce polypharmacy, and improve drug management with pharmacists and healthcare professionals.

Psychosocial Factors in Rehabilitative Practices:

Psychosocial factors are very important in rehabilitation and have a big influence on the health and results of patients. A few things to think about are:

Provide emotional and psychological support to individuals dealing with accident, disability, or chronic illness. Offer patients services, support groups, and therapy to assist them deal with stress, anxiety, depression, and adjusting to life transitions.

Patient Motivation and Engagement: To design interventions that encourage active participation and engagement in rehabilitation, it is important to understand the patient's objectives, values, and motivations. To empower patients and promote self-efficacy, employ motivational interviewing approaches.

Social Support: Acknowledge the significance of social support systems, such as friends, family, caregivers, and local resources, in the healing process. To improve patient outcomes, include support systems in the planning, goal-setting, and decision-making processes.

Cultural Sensitivity: When it comes to rehabilitation, respect cultural values, beliefs, and preferences. Take into account cultural aspects that could impact the patient's treatment preferences, attitudes toward disabilities, and health beliefs, and modify interventions as necessary.

Healthcare professionals can provide patient-centered treatment that fits the individual needs and preferences of people of all ages by taking special concerns in rehabilitation into account. This will improve outcomes and foster overall well-being. Providing thorough and efficient rehabilitation services to a variety of patient demographics requires teamwork, communication, and empathy.

THE END

www.ingramcontent.com/pod-product-compliance
Lightning Source LLC
Chambersburg PA
CBHW070157230526
45471CB00002B/696